OVERCOMING DEPRESSION:

A SIMPLE WAY TO FEELING BETTER

KAREN WESLEY Ph.D

Depression is a typical and crippling temperament issue. Something beyond misery in light of life's battles and misfortunes, gloom changes how you think, feel, and capacity in day by day exercises. It can meddle with your capacity to work, think about, eat, rest, and appreciate life. The sentiments of vulnerability, misery, and uselessness can be exceptional and tenacious, with little, assuming any, help.

While a few people depict sadness as "living in a dark gap" or having a sentiment of approaching fate, others feel inert, unfilled, and impassive. Depression frequently shifts as per age and sexual orientation, with side effects varying among people, or youngsters and more seasoned grown-ups. Loss of energy, sleep changes, loss of interest are some of the symptoms of depression.

Contents

CHAPTER ONE 1

WHAT IS DEPRESSION? 1

SIDE EFFECTS 2

CHAPTER TWO 7

DEPRESSION EFFECTS AMONG VARIOUS PEOPLE 7

TALK TO SOMEONE 13

CHAPTER THREE 15

WHAT CAUSES DEPRESSION? 15

CHAPTER FOUR 26

DEPRESSION: HELPING A FAMILY MEMBER OR A FRIEND 26

THIS IS WHAT YOU CAN DO HELP:.. 32

THINK ABOUT THESE ISSUES: 35

CHAPTER ONE

WHAT IS DEPRESSION?

Depression is a state of mind issue that causes a tenacious sentiment of trouble and loss of intrigue. Additionally called significant burdensome issue or clinical despondency, it influences how you feel, think and carry on and can prompt an assortment of enthusiastic and physical issues. You may experience difficulty doing typical everyday exercises, and now and again you may feel as though life does not merit living.

Something beyond an episode of the blues, melancholy isn't a shortcoming and you can't just "snap out" of it. Sadness may require long haul treatment. However, don't get disheartened. A great many people with misery feel better with drug, psychotherapy or both.

SIDE EFFECTS
In spite of the fact that wretchedness may happen just once amid your life, individuals normally have different scenes. Amid these scenes, manifestations happen the

greater part of the day, consistently and may include:

- Sentiments of trouble, sorrow, void or sadness
- Irate upheavals, crabbiness or dissatisfaction, even over little issues
- Loss of intrigue or joy in most or every ordinary action, for example, sex, side interests or sports
- Rest unsettling influences, including a sleeping disorder or dozing excessively

- Tiredness and absence of vitality, so even little undertakings require additional exertion
- Diminished hunger and weight reduction or expanded yearnings for nourishment and weight gain
- Tension, disturbance or eagerness
- Hindered thinking, talking or body developments

- Sentiments of uselessness or blame, focusing on past disappointments or self-fault
- Inconvenience thinking, concentrating, settling on choices and recollecting things
- Visit or intermittent considerations of death, self-destructive contemplations, suicide endeavors or suicide
- Unexplained physical issues, for example, back agony or cerebral pains

For some individuals with sadness, side effects for the most part are extreme enough to make perceptible issues in day exercises, for example, work, school, social exercises or associations with others. A few people may feel commonly hopeless or troubled without truly knowing why.

CHAPTER TWO

DEPRESSION EFFECTS AMONG VARIOUS PEOPLE

Misery side effects in kids and teenagers

Basic signs and side effects of sorrow in youngsters and adolescents are like those of grown-ups; however there can be a few contrasts.

In more youthful youngsters, side effects of sorrow may incorporate trouble, fractiousness, clinginess, stress, a throbbing painfulness, declining to go to class, or being underweight.

In teenagers, side effects may incorporate pity, crabbiness, feeling negative and useless, outrage, poor execution or poor participation at school, feeling misconstrued and amazingly delicate, utilizing recreational medications or liquor, eating or resting excessively, self-hurt, loss of enthusiasm for ordinary exercises, and shirking of social collaboration.

Gloom side effects in more seasoned grown-ups

Gloom is certainly not an ordinary piece of becoming more established, and it ought to never be trifled with. Sadly, dejection frequently goes undiscovered and untreated in more established grown-ups, and they may feel hesitant to look for assistance. Indications of melancholy might be unique or more subtle in more seasoned grown-ups, for example,

Memory troubles or character changes

Physical throbs or agony

Exhaustion, loss of craving, rest issues or loss of enthusiasm for sex — not brought about by an ailment or medicine

Frequently needing to remain at home, as opposed to going out to mingle or doing new things

Self-destructive reasoning or emotions, particularly in more seasoned men

At the point when to see a specialist

In the event that you feel discouraged, make an arrangement to see your specialist or psychological well-being proficient when you can. In case you're hesitant to look for treatment, converse with a companion or cherished one, any medicinal services proficient, a confidence head, or another person you trust.

At the point when to get crisis help

In the event that you figure you may hurt yourself or endeavor suicide, call 911 or your neighborhood crisis number right away.

Likewise consider these alternatives in case you're having self-destructive contemplations:

TALK TO SOMEONE

Call your specialist or psychological well-being proficient.

Call a suicide hotline number — in the U.S., call the National Suicide Prevention Lifeline at 1-800-273-TALK (1-800-273-8255). Utilize that equivalent number and press "1" to achieve the Veterans Crisis Line.

Connect with a dear companion or cherished one.

Contact a clergyman, otherworldly pioneer or another person in your confidence network.

In the event that you have a friend or family member who is in threat of suicide or has made a suicide endeavor, ensure somebody remains with that individual. Call 911 or your nearby crisis number right away. Or on the other hand, in the event that you want to do as such securely, take the individual to the closest clinic crisis room.

CHAPTER THREE

WHAT CAUSES DEPRESSION?

It's not known precisely what causes misery. Likewise with numerous psychological issue, an assortment of components might be included, for example,

- Organic contrasts. Individuals with sadness seem to have physical changes in their cerebrums. The noteworthiness of these progressions is as yet questionable, yet may in the end help pinpoint causes.

- Mind science. Synapses are normally happening mind synthetic concoctions that possible assume a job in discouragement. Ongoing exploration shows that adjustments in the capacity and impact of these synapses and how they communicate with neurocircuits associated with keeping up state of mind steadiness may assume a critical job in gloom and its treatment.

- Hormones. Changes in the body's parity of hormones might be engaged with causing or activating despondency. Hormone changes can result with pregnancy and amid the weeks or months after conveyance (baby blues) and from thyroid issues, menopause or various different conditions.

- Acquired attributes. Wretchedness is increasingly basic in individuals whose blood relatives likewise have this condition. Scientists are attempting to discover qualities that might be engaged with causing gloom.

- Hazard factors

Sadness frequently starts in the youngsters, 20s or 30s, yet it can occur at any age. A greater number of ladies than men are determined to have despondency, yet this might be expected to a limited extent since ladies are bound to look for treatment.

Components that appear to expand the danger of creating or activating discouragement include:

Certain character qualities, for example, low confidence and being excessively needy, self-basic or cynical

Awful or upsetting occasions, for example, physical or sexual maltreatment, the demise or loss of a friend or family member, a troublesome relationship, or budgetary issues

Blood relatives with a background marked by misery, bipolar confusion, liquor addiction or suicide

Being lesbian, gay, indiscriminate or transgender, or having varieties in the improvement of genital organs that aren't unmistakably male or female (intersex) in an unsupportive circumstance

History of other emotional wellness issue, for example, nervousness issue, dietary problems or post-awful pressure issue

Maltreatment of liquor or recreational medications

Genuine or endless ailment, including malignancy, stroke, incessant agony or coronary illness

Certain prescriptions, for example, some hypertension drugs or dozing pills (converse with your specialist before halting any medicine)

Confusions

Discouragement is a genuine issue that can negatively affect you and your family. Sadness regularly deteriorates on the off chance that it isn't dealt with, bringing about passionate, social and medical issues that influence each aspect of your life.

Instances of difficulties related with sorrow include:

Abundance weight or heftiness, which can prompt coronary illness and diabetes

Torment or physical ailment

Liquor or medication abuse

Nervousness, alarm issue or social fear

Family clashes, relationship troubles, and work or school issues

Social segregation

Self-destructive sentiments, suicide endeavors or suicide

Self-mutilation, for example, cutting

Unexpected passing from ailments

Counteractive action

There's no certain method to counteract misery. Nonetheless, these techniques may help.

Find a way to control worry, to expand your versatility and lift your confidence.

Connect with family and companions, particularly in the midst of emergency, to enable you to climate unpleasant spells.

Get treatment at the soonest indication of an issue to help keep sadness from exacerbating.

Consider getting long haul support treatment to help forestall a backslide of side effects.

CHAPTER FOUR

DEPRESSION: HELPING A FAMILY MEMBER OR A FRIEND

Helping somebody with depression can be a test. In the event that somebody in your life has gloom, you may feel defenseless and wonder what to do. Figure out how to offer help and comprehension and how to enable your cherished one to get the assets to adapt to sorrow. This is what you can do.

Become familiar with the side effects of depression

Melancholy signs and side effects change from individual to individual. They can include:

Sentiments of trouble, mournfulness, void or sadness

Irate upheavals, touchiness or dissatisfaction, even over little issues

Loss of intrigue or delight in most or every single ordinary action, for example, sex, interests or sports

A sleeping disorder or resting excessively

Tiredness and absence of vitality, so even little errands require additional exertion

Changes in hunger — decreased hunger and weight reduction or expanded desires for nourishment and weight gain

Tension, tumult or anxiety

Hindered thinking, talking or body developments

Sentiments of uselessness or blame, focusing on past disappointments or reprimanding yourself for things that aren't your obligation

Inconvenience thinking, concentrating, settling on choices and recollecting things

Continuous or intermittent notice of death, self-destructive considerations, suicide endeavors or suicide

Unexplained physical issues, for example, back torment or cerebral pains

For some individuals with gloom, indications for the most part are sufficiently serious to make observable issues in day exercises, for example, work, school, social exercises or associations with others. Other individuals may feel commonly hopeless or troubled without knowing why. Youngsters and teenagers may demonstrate melancholy by being bad tempered or irritable as opposed to miserable.

Energize treatment

Individuals with gloom may not perceive or recognize that they're discouraged. They may not know about signs and indications of gloom, so they may think their emotions are typical.

Very frequently, individuals feel embarrassed about their discouragement and erroneously trust they ought to have the option to defeat it with self discipline alone. In any case, sadness only here and there shows signs of improvement without treatment and may deteriorate. With the correct treatment approach, the individual you care about can show signs of improvement.

THIS IS WHAT YOU CAN DO TO HELP:
- Converse with the individual about what you've seen and for what reason you're concerned.
- Clarify that sadness is an ailment, not an individual imperfection or shortcoming — and that it typically shows

signs of improvement with treatment.

- Recommend looking for assistance from an expert — a therapeutic specialist or a psychological well-being supplier, for example, an authorized advisor or analyst.
- Offer to help set up a rundown of inquiries to examine in an underlying meeting with a specialist or emotional wellness supplier.
- Express your eagerness to help by setting up arrangements, coming to

them and going to family treatment sessions.
- On the off chance that your cherished one's ailment is extreme or conceivably hazardous, contact a specialist, a clinic or crisis therapeutic administrations.
- Recognize cautioning indications of exacerbating sorrow

Everybody encounters despondency in an unexpected way. Watch your adored one. Figure out how sorrow influences your relative or companion — and realize what to do when it deteriorates.

THINK ABOUT THESE ISSUES:

- What are the run of the mill signs and side effects of discouragement in your relative or companion?
- What practices or language do you see when sadness is more regrettable?

- What practices or language do you see when the individual is progressing nicely?
- What conditions trigger scenes of progressively extreme gloom?
- What exercises are most useful when misery intensifies?

Intensifying misery should be treated as quickly as time permits. Urge your adored one to work with his or her specialist or emotional wellness supplier to concoct an arrangement for what to do when signs and side effects achieve a specific point. As a component of this arrangement, your cherished one may need to:

- Contact the specialist to see about altering or changing drugs
- See a psychotherapist, for example, an authorized advocate or therapist
- Make self-care strides, for example, being certain to eat well suppers, get a fitting

measure of rest and be physically dynamic
- Comprehend suicide hazard

Individuals with discouragement are at an expanded danger of suicide. In the event that your adored one is seriously discouraged, set yourself up for the likelihood that sooner or later the individual in question may feel self-destructive. Pay attention to all indications of self-destructive conduct and act right away.

www.ingramcontent.com/pod-product-compliance
Lightning Source LLC
Chambersburg PA
CBHW030541220526
45463CB00007B/2929